Habit Building for Introverts

A Guide to Thriving in an Extroverted World

Norman F. Norman

Table of Contents

The monotony and solitude of a quiet life stimulates the creative mind.

— Albert Einstein

Chapter 1. Introduction

Welcome to the exciting journey of habit-building tailor-made for the introverts amongst us! Our Special Report, "Habit Building for Introverts: A Guide to Thriving in an Extroverted World," illuminates the fascinating world of introversion and notably, how to navigate it with confidence and success. This is not your everyday guide; it's specially crafted with insightful strategies, intuitive solutions, and empowering habits designed to help you not just survive, but truly thrive in our extrovert-dominated society. Bursting with easy-to-understand concepts and practical tips, our guide paints a vivid map for introverts seeking to harness their unique strengths. Grab your copy now and set off on this transformative journey- because this world needs the power of your quiet strength!

Chapter 2. Understanding Introversion: Beyond the Stereotypes

Introversion, often misunderstood and labeled with stereotypes, is a far more complex concept than is commonly assumed. It goes beyond the simple definition of being shy or reserved; it's about where one gets their energy and how they process the world around them. Buckle up and get ready to unravel the rich tapestry of introversion, dispelling the stereotypes, and embracing the inherent strengths that lie within.

2.1. The Essence of Introversion

Introverts, in the most rudimentary form, are individuals who feel energized in solitude and quiet surroundings, in contrast with extroverts who draw energy from social interactions. However, it is a spectrum with varying degrees, complexities, and subtleties. Surely, it's not about being entirely antisocial or having a dislike for human company; it's rather a preference for a different kind of interaction.

Introverts often process information internally, delve deeper into thoughts, and exhibit higher sensitivity to external stimuli. They set their joy's tempo by indulging in introspection, imagination, and incubation of ideas. They relish vibrant mindscape fuelled by thoughts, ideas, reflections, and often, profound, meaningful one-on-one conversations.

2.2. The Introversion-Extroversion Spectrum

Contrary to popular belief, introversion and extroversion are not binaries. They're endpoints on a spectrum, also known as the introversion-extroversion continuum. You may imagine this line starting from extreme introversion, passing through ambiversion, and ending with extreme extroversion.

Psychologist Carl Jung, who first popularized these terms, emphasized that no one is a pure introvert or pure extrovert. Instead, most people oscillate between these two points, with a natural inclination towards one end. This spectrum helps us understand the nuanced nature of our personalities, making space for variations and fluidity.

2.3. The Brain Science Behind Introversion

The disparity between introverts and extroverts lies deep within our neurological system. Scientific research shows that the brain chemicals dopamine and acetylcholine play crucial roles.

While dopamine is a neurotransmitter associated with reward-seeking behaviors, external stimuli, and instant gratification, Acetylcholine is linked with pleasure related to introspection, long-term planning, and focus. The brains of introverts prefer the slow, steady burn of acetylcholine, as opposed to the dopamine high for extroverts.

Further, the introvert's brain follows a different dominant pathway for processing stimuli. It passes through areas associated with remembering, planning, and problem-solving, implying a more internalized processing and response to external stimuli.

2.4. Debunking Common Stereotypes

Now, let's debunk some prevalent stereotypes surrounding introversion:

1. **Myth: Introverts are antisocial or shy.** Fact: Introversion isn't synonymous with shyness or antisocial behavior. Introverts can be sociable and possess impressive people skills but prefer deep, meaningful interactions, and often require downtime after social events.

2. **Myth: Introverts don't make good leaders or public speakers.** Fact: Given their propensity for thoughtful decision-making and active listening, introverts can be exceptional leaders. As speakers, their powerful insights often shine through, giving rise to compelling narratives.

3. **Myth: Introverts always want to be alone.** Fact: While solitude is vital for their emotional replenishment, introverts do appreciate meaningful human connection. What matters to them is the quality, not quantity, of their social interactions.

By better understanding introversion and dispeling these myths, society can begin to appreciate the depth, insightfulness, and quiet energy brought by those with an introverted disposition.

2.5. Embracing Your Introversion

Recognizing and accepting your introversion is the first step towards leveraging it to your advantage. You possess unique strengths – deep-rooted empathy, reflective thinking, careful decision-making, and more. Cherish these qualities, for they set you apart in this loud world. Allowing introverted traits to shine through your work and relationships paves the way for authentic, purpose-driven lives, breaking free from societal molds.

This chapter aimed to unravel the complexities behind introversion, scratching the societal stereotypes' surface. However, remember that introversion is not a one-size-fits-all label. It's a spectrum, and everyone's experience with it is unique. Use this knowledge as your compass to better understand yourself, leverage your strengths, and debunk the common stereotypes associated with introversive personality traits.

As we advance towards realizing the power of introversion, remember to embrace it wholeheartedly. Be patient with yourself, acknowledging this is just the beginning of a more profound journey into self-acceptance and actualization. So sit back, relax, and let's delve into the rest of this exciting journey in the following chapters.

In the next chapters, we will focus on accepting your personality traits, honing your latent potential, creating beneficial habits for personal growth, and successfully navigating the world dominated by an 'extrovert ideal'.

Chapter 3. Accepting Your Introversion: The Power Within You

In this enlightening journey, we will delve into the depths of accepting introversion, ultimately unearthing the dormant strength residing within each introvert. The essence of embracing your identity flows from understanding and acceptance - and then utilizing those revelations for personal development. The power within you - your introverted nature - is not a shortcoming to be hidden, but, quite the contrary, a wellspring of unique strengths poised to take you on a path of growth, if harnessed correctly.

3.1. Understanding Your True Nature

Let us first address the elephant in the room: what does it mean to be an introvert? Contrary to popular stereotyping, introversion does not equate to being socially awkward or perpetually shy. Introversion, in simple terms, involves deriving energy from solitude and processing experiences internally. You see, introverts possess the ability to turn inwards, drawing strength from within, rather than relying on external stimulation. What a fascinating, self-sustaining ecosystem they harbor!

Introversion should not be perceived as a liability; it's an integral part of your personality, one that you should accept with open arms. Available literature on Carl Jung's work provides compelling evidence that both introversion and extraversion fall on a spectrum; they aren't monoliths but fluid constructs. Hence, accepting your introversion doesn't mean shunning extraverted tendencies, only acknowledging where you typically derive energy from.

3.2. Embracing Your Introversion: Tap into Your Inner Power

The first step to harnessing your inner power involves self-acceptance. Casually disregarding your introverted nature does not change it; instead, it raises self-doubt and fosters anxiety. Understand this: there's an abundant source of power within you, shaping your holistic identity and the unique manner through which you perceive the world.

An introvert's vivid inner world enables profound insight, promotes creativity, reinforces empathy, and augments analytical prowess – traits that can be transformed into personal superpowers, once acknowledged and nurtured. Embrace this evidence of your innate potential, for in the acceptance of your individuality lies immense personal fulfillment and growth.

3.3. Building Confidence: Celebrate Your Individuality

Your introverted nature should be a cause of celebration, not condemnation. Indeed, in a world that often fixates on extroverted traits, such as social prowess and outgoing nature, being an introvert might sometimes feel like a square peg trying to fit into a round hole. But remember this: your individuality should always be your strength, not your weak point. Susan Cain, in her book 'Quiet: The Power of Introverts in a World That Can't Stop Talking,' underlines the importance of introverts in various walks of life.

Introverts often play the essential role of thoughtful leaders, empathetic team members, and creative thinkers. Furthermore, they excel in independent work and show stellar performance in roles that demand innovative problem-solving strategies. You should be proud of your introverted nature and ride the wave of your individuality to construct a solid foundation of self-confidence.

3.4. Turning Challenges into Strengths: The Introvert's Guide

Constructing an understanding of oneself and learning to accept our intrinsic traits can sometimes present a challenge, especially when these characteristics are perceived as different or unorthodox by societal norms. Nevertheless, as an introvert, the ability to look beyond these externally imposed limitations can help transform these challenges into personal advantages and strengths.

A common misconception is that introverts lack social skills, but the reality is that introverts simply approach social scenarios differently. Introverts are renowned for their listening skills, depth in conversation, and excellent observation, which in many circumstances, are far more beneficial than superficial chit-chat. To leverage these inherent capabilities, focus on quality over quantity; prioritize meaningful relationships and stimulating conversations over casual social flutters.

3.5. Conclusion: The Power Within You

Accepting your introversion is the first step towards harnessing your inner power and turning it into a beacon of personal strength. By embracing the unique characteristics of your introverted nature, understanding their implications, and seeking ways to use these qualities to your advantage, you can not only survive but flourish in a world that seems tilted towards extroversion. The power within you, as an introvert, is immense and unique, overflowing with potential to enhance personal growth, career opportunities, and social interactions. Embrace your introversion, and let your quiet strength guide your path to success, happiness, and fulfillment. That is the quintessential power within you, and it's about time the world witnesses its sheer magnitude and brilliance.

Chapter 4. Thriving as an Introvert: Outlining the Strategies

In this uniquitous voyage through the empowering domain of introversion, we cease our engines at the critical juncture of strategies which, when skilfully implemented, can facilitate thriving as an introvert. This chapter will meticulously delve into tactical manoeuvres that can harness introverts' greatest strengths and readily equip them with the tools necessary to succeed in an extroverted world.

4.1. The Power In The Pause

Let's embark on this exploration by first understanding the infinite strength of silence, of pausing. Introverts possess a dominant trait - they are reflective thinkers. They tend to contemplate before speaking, exuding thoughtfulness and depth. Using this to your advantage is crucial: that pause, that moment of silence before you speak, can be a beacon of respect and contemplation in the noise of the extroverted world. It refines the quality of your conversation, steering it towards meaningful interactions rather than surface-level discourse.

4.2. Deep Dive: Focus and Concentration

Introverts exhibit a remarkable ability to concentrate and focus on tasks at hand. Running in the mostly singular track of thought, introverts excel at diving deep into subjects, exploring various layers and complexities. This trait can be leveraged to acquire profound knowledge, exhibit expertise in specialized fields, and establish credibility. By deploying your capacity to concentrate, introverts can thrive in projects that require meticulousness, accuracy, and an eye for detail.

4.3. The Art of Solo Productivity

The inclination towards solitude, often mistaken as a weakness, is, in fact, one of the most potent strengths of an introvert. Leveraging solitude for productivity can yield excellent results. The stillness and quietude can become the breeding grounds for creativity, innovation, and problem-solving. Spaces devoid of external interruptions provide fertile ground for the nurturing of ideas and concepts, leading to abundant productivity.

4.4. The Strength of Active Listening

Often, extroverts are praised for their communication prowess, but effective communication doesn't solely rely on eloquent speech. A significant part is listening, an art in which introverts naturally excel. Active listening allows a thorough understanding of ideas and displays empathy and respect toward the speaker. Emphasizing this attribute can augment team dynamics, foster stronger relationships, and, crucially, can place introverts as potent problem solvers.

4.5. Preferred Modes of Communication

Most introverts are known to express themselves better in written format. Harnessing this to your advantage can open new avenues in personal and professional domains. Writing enables deliberate thought, aids clarity, and allows the freedom of time and space. Be it emails, reports, or textual conversations, introverts can leverage their written communication skills to make a significant impact.

4.6. Building Meaningful Relationships

Unlike extroverts who prefer an extensive network, introverts naturally drift towards building a few but in-depth and meaningful relationships. Over time, these relationships prove quite fruitful, providing a support system and fostering growth in various aspects of life. Nurturing these relationships by investing quality time and effort can significantly enhance personal and professional spheres.

4.7. Finding Your Quiet Courage

Contrary to the prevailing norms, courage does not always roar. Sometimes, it is the quiet voice at the end of the day affirming that you will try again tomorrow. As an introvert, your quiet courage is the rock upon which you build your foundation of strength. It's the gentle force propelling you forward. Recognizing and nurturing this quiet courage is crucial.

This chapter illuminates the potential pathways for introverts to flourish in their unique ways. The power lies not in seeking to transform into an extrovert but in embracing the introverted traits and channeling them to your advantage. A strategic approach, as we have seen above, can chart a course for success and fulfillment for any introvert in an extroverted world.

Remember, the world may be loud, but that does not mean you have to compete with the noise. Within you lies a quiet strength of immense value - your introverted traits. By harnessing these, you can leave an impactful, lasting imprint in your personal and professional life. The world needs the distinct strengths you bring to the table. It's time to stimulate your strategic thinking. Let's outline the success story of "you, the introvert," align your inherent traits with the operational dynamics of this world, and forge a path distinctly your own.

Chapter 5. Building Beneficial Habits: A Step-By-Step Guide

Habit building is a technique that has been revered in the personal development scene for years, arguably centuries. We'll start by exploring why it's so important, providing a substantial, research-backed foundation for our subsequent advice. Following that, we will delve into some tailored strategies for introverts looking to develop beneficial habits and conclude with some very specific methods and practices based on common scenarios and challenges facing introverts today.

5.1. Significance of Habit Building

Habits are the subconscious patterns of behavior we engage in on a daily basis. These habits can be manual, like tying our shoelaces or brushing our teeth, and they can also be mental, like reassessing our decisions or thinking critically about the information we receive. Habits shape our lives in significant ways, and this is found throughout literature, science, and philosophy.

James Clear, the author of Atomic Habits, makes a compelling case for the power of habits. "Habits are the compound interest of self-improvement," Clear asserts. This analogy is striking and impactful in its simplicity. Just as your money grows exponentially with compound interest, so does the effect of your habits on your life.

Charles Duhigg, in his book The Power of Habit, argues that habits function in a three-step loop: Cue, Routine, and Reward. The Cue triggers the habit, the Routine involves the actions you take, and the Reward is the benefit you gain from acting out the habit. Recognizing and understanding these elements can prove to be a powerful lever in effectively building beneficial habits.

5.2. Introverts and Habits

While everyone can benefit from good habits, it's important to understand that being an introvert can sometimes add a layer of complexity to the process of habit formation. Since introverts tend to derive energy from within and can feel drained by excessive social interaction, it's important that the habits they build align with their innate tendencies.

Learning to recognize and respect your personal energy levels and triggers should be a fundamental starting point. This can form the basis of habits designed to amplify your strengths and manage your energy effectively.

Introverts often shine in areas where deep focus and thought are required. Therefore, habits that promote these strengths - such as creating quiet, alone time for contemplation and creating regular routines for deep work - can be particularly beneficial.

5.3. Step-by-step Guide to Building Habits for Introverts

Now that we understand the why, let's delve into the how. The process of forming new habits can be broken down into several, manageable steps. This guide is designed to help you navigate this process as an introvert.

Step 1: Awareness The first step in building a habit is to recognize your current habits. Duhigg recommends keeping a habit journal where you describe the Cue, Routine, and Reward for each habit. For introverts, make sure to include habits relating to how you handle social interactions and manage your energy.

Step 2: Define your Core Habits Consider the energy management strategies that work well for you. Maybe you need quiet mornings to start your day or a brief solitude break in the afternoon. Once you've identified these strategies, you can build them into your core habits.

Step 3: Start Small James Clear advocates beginning with small actions. Select a habit that's so simple it seems too straightforward to fail. For example, if quiet reflection time is a core habit, start by dedicating just five minutes a day.

Step 4: Be Consistent Consistency is more important than perfection. Ensure you're performing your new habits regularly. Sticking to regular patterns and routines can be especially comforting for introverts.

Step 5: Leverage Existing Habits Known as habit stacking, Duhigg suggests attaching new habits to existing ones, making the new behavior more likely to stick. For example, you might spend five minutes in quiet reflection during your regular morning coffee routine.

5.4. Practical Habits that Benefit Introverts

To end this chapter, let's discuss some practical habits that have proven particularly advantageous for introverts.

Habit 1: Set Boundaries Introverts thrive when they have personal space and time. It's essential to build boundaries in your professional as well as personal life. Learn to say "no", delegate tasks when necessary, and avoid overextending yourself socially.

Habit 2: Cultivate Alone Time Whether it's through reading, walking in nature, or practicing mindfulness, make sure to dedicate time for just you. This habit can help introverts recharge and gain clarity.

Habit 3: Practice Mindful Socializing You don't have to avoid social scenarios altogether, but practice mindful socializing. Choose quality over quantity. Opt for deep, meaningful connections rather than superficial small talks.

In sum, always remember that being an introvert is not a disadvantage. Your quiet strength and thoughtful approach can be beneficial not only to you but also to the people around you. But leveraging these strengths often requires developing habits that play to your strengths and mitigate potential areas of struggle. And this chapter is a comprehensive guide on how to do exactly that.

Chapter 6. Introvert Energy Management: Maximizing Your Potential

Many individuals underestimate the importance of energy management, often focusing instead on time management. This short-sighted approach, especially among introverts, fails to take into account the unique way in which they experience and harness their energy. This chapter dives deeply into the concept of Introvert Energy Management, offering intricate details about its significance, the science behind it, the challenges associated with it, and how to efficiently maximize your potential energy.

6.1. Anchoring your Energy: Understanding the Dynamics

Before we explore the methods of managing and maximizing introvert energy, it is crucial to comprehend the mechanism that underlies it. Introverts, unlike extroverts, derive and replenish their energy reservoir in solace, often feeling drained in highly stimulative environments. This characteristic trait of introverts is rooted in their neurobiology, where the 'Dopamine' and 'Acetylcholine' pathways play prominent roles. While extroverts thrive on dopamine, a neurotransmitter that stimulates the reward and pleasure pathways of our brains in response to social interaction, introverts lean more toward acetylcholine, which fuels our reflective and contemplative states. Hence, understanding these dynamics forms the foundation for effective energy management.

6.2. The Art of Energy Conservation

Due emphasis should be laid on the art of energy conservation as an integral part of energy management. Unlike the traditional approach, which emphasizes engaging in more activities for energy utilization, an inquiry into energy conservation lends the opportunity to observe and align your activities with natural energy levels. Mindfully approach situations that could potentially be energy draining. Consider, for instance, scheduling necessary social engagements for times when your energy is naturally higher, or limiting exposure to crowded environments that tend to drain your energy reserves. Inclusive of habits like prioritizing personal time, regular periods of quiet reflection, and stress management through activities like meditative rituals and yoga, the art of energy conservation acts as a fitting buffer against energy drain.

6.3. Charting Your Energy Timeline: Finding Your Unique Rhythm

An effective strategy for enacting energy management is charting your energy timeline. This involves identifying periods throughout the day when your energy levels naturally fluctuate. It requires mindful observation and patience as energy patterns may not always follow a linear or predictable course. The goal is to coincide high-energy periods with demanding activities and reserve low-energy periods for restful and rejuvenating practices. Moreover, this timeline should stay flexible, adapting to changes in daily schedules or situational demands.

6.4. Techniques for Energy Replenishment

Acknowledging the inevitable instances of energy depletion, our focus should also concentrate on techniques for prompt and efficient energy replenishment. Introverts typically recharge their energy stores in solitude and indulging in low-stimulus activities. The solitude sought by introverts may come in several forms, such as a quiet walk in nature, reading a favorite book, or enjoying a personal hobby. Recharging one's introvert batteries could also include deep, meaningful one-on-one conversations, contradicting the common misconception that introverts prefer absolute solitude. Furthermore, adequate sleep, proper nutrition, and regular physical activity have been scientifically proven to boost overall energy levels. Thus, incorporating these components in your routine is highly recommended.

6.5. The Role of Self-Acceptance and Self-Care

At the core of introvert energy management lies the practice of self-acceptance and self-care. In a world that tends to facilitate and reward extroverted behavior, introverts might sometimes feel pressured to act against their natural disposition, leading to significant energy drain and emotional strain. Recognizing and accepting your introverted nature, therefore, remains a crucial aspect of managing your energy. Similarly, regularly practicing self-care, such as setting boundaries, taking mental health days, or simply enjoying some 'alone time', demonstrate essential ways to prioritize yourself and your energy needs.

6.6. Customizing Your Environment: Spatial energy dynamics

Lastly, tailoring your environment to suit your energy needs can do wonders for managing your energy levels. Spatial energy dynamics are a seldom explored but potent concept. Creating personal sanctuaries at home or office, limiting exposure to unnecessary visual or auditory stimuli, and using colors, light, and décor to evoke tranquility, can subtly nurture your introvert energy.

In conclusion, Introvert Energy Management is a multidimensional concept that emphasizes the importance of understanding, conserving, and replenishing your energy. The mentioned strategies and techniques all aim to build an encompassing view towards managing energy effectively. By accepting your introverted nature, recognizing your unique energy rhythm, and making necessary adaptations in your life, you can truly maximize your potential in an extroverted world. The journey may require patience and commitment but remember, in the stillness often lies the power. Lean into it.

Chapter 7. Coping with Social Pressure: Tools for Resilience

The realm of social interaction, filled with nuanced complexities, has often proven to be a major challenge for introverts, whether it be at work, in interpersonal relationships, or in general social scenarios. However, this chapter aims to delve into enriching strategies and practical tools that introverts can deploy to cope with social pressure and build resilience. While we acknowledge that social scenarios can sometimes feel like an insurmountable hurdle, we seek to furnish you with an arsenal of tools to not just evade, but navigate through these instances with newfound strength and resilience. This write-up is well-rounded and exhaustive, aimed at unpacking numerous tools and strategies to cope with social pressure.

7.1. Psychological Tools for Resilience

An introvert's first line of defense against social pressure are psychological tools. Techniques like cognitive reframing, mindfulness, and positive affirmations can grant introverts the fortitude to endure social pressure. Cognitive reframing encourages you to alter your perception of a stressful event, transforming it from a threat to a challenge. This perspective change can significantly alleviate perceived social pressure. Pairing cognitive reframing with mindfulness, the conscious process of maintaining awareness of our thoughts, feelings, and surroundings, can further enhance your psychological resilience.

Positive affirmations, which involve the use of uplifting and encouraging statements, can reframe your mindset to a more constructive one, boosting your self-esteem and combating negative self-talk often associated with social pressure. Introverts struggling with social pressure can use affirmations such as "I am capable of handling any social situation that comes my way" or "I am comfortable in my introversion." These affirmations serve as a psychological shield against adversity, fortifying your mental resilience.

7.2. Building and Maintaining Energy Reserves

For introverts, social situations can be powerfully draining. Recharging and building energy reserves are therefore crucial. Introverts should prioritize regular intervals of silence or solitude to recharge and restore their energy levels. Creative outlets like art, writing, or playing an instrument can also be used as recuperative activities. Engage in regular exercise, ensure adequate sleep, and maintain a nutritious diet, helping your body to physically cope with stress triggered by social pressure.

7.3. Developing Communication Skills

Effective communication can dramatically lessen the anxiety attached to social encounters. One working strategy is to initially focus on one-on-one or small group interactions rather than large gatherings. Introverts often excel in these settings, as they tend to foster deeper, more meaningful conversations. Practice active listening, a skill that involves fully focusing on, comprehending, and responding to a speaker. This silent back-and-forth can provide breathing space in social gatherings and turn conversation into a more manageable activity.

7.4. Building Relationships: From Strangers to Acquaintances

Another important strategy for handling social pressure is to gradually cultivate closer relationships, starting from acquaintances. The transition from stranger to acquaintance can lessen the pressure that comes with unknown territory. Developing relationships also calls for intricacies like understanding body language, gauging mood, and reciprocating conversation, all of which, with practice, can enhance your social comfort.

7.5. Embracing Imperfection and Courageous Self-expression

Learning to embrace imperfection is arguably one of the most daunting, yet transformational facets of overcoming social pressure. Acknowledging that occasional social faux pas are just part of the journey can be liberating. Embrace assertiveness and express your needs confidently without fear of criticism or rejection. This assertive self-expression not only fosters self-respect but also builds resilience against social pressure.

While these tools and strategies provide a roadmap for introverts to navigate social pressure, remember that effective change is gradual and requires consistent effort. With time, patience, and practice, you can turn these strategies into daily habits that empower you to deal effectively with social pressures, nurturing the confident, resilient introvert within you.

Chapter 8. Introverted Leadership: Shaping Your Unique Path

Many have been conditioned to believe that leadership is synonymous with extroversion. It's a misconception deeply ingrained in our societal fabric, seeded by misunderstandings of introversion and propagated by an extroverted view of what it means to lead. In this chapter, we delve into the core essence of introverted leadership and how to shape your unique path as an introverted leader.

8.1. The Misunderstood Introverted Leader

There's a popular yet misinterpreted image of leaders: they're always outgoing, boisterous, and can command a room with booming voices and charisma. However, this perception shuns the reality where many impactful leaders exhibit introverted qualities. Introverted leaders are highly contemplative, deep thinkers, excellent listeners, and usually have the ability to connect on a one-to-one basis—a quality that distinctively separates them from their extroverted counterparts.

With the ability to listen before speaking, introverted leaders often gain an in-depth understanding of situations, which aids in productive decision making. Equal part observers and deep thinkers, they prefer to fully work through ideas alone before presenting them to the team—thus, ensuring that the concepts are thoughtfully evaluated and represent well-rounded perspectives.

8.2. Embracing Your Leadership Style

As an introverted leader, it is crucial to recognize and embrace your distinctive style and leverage it to your advantage. You are a leader blessed with the power of deep reflections, enabling you to provide insightful directions and conclusions.

Introverted leaders often display considerable emotional intelligence. This quality means that you're likely attuned to your team's feelings and are more empathetic. You can leverage this to create an environment that encourages open communication and fosters high morale.

Remember, there is no one-size-fits-all method to leadership. Leadership is not limited to extroverted traits — it's about making the most of your inherent strengths and utilizing them to lead effectively.

8.3. Harnessing Your Strengths

Having understood the unique traits of an introverted leader, you must learn to harness these to your advantage. Here are some steps:

- Practice active listening: Ensure everyone in your team feels heard and valued by making active listening a priority. Receive feedback graciously and create a supportive environment for employees to share their thoughts and concerns.

- Use thoughtful communication: Choose your words carefully to provide clear instructions and avoid misunderstandings. Your ability to reflect and think deeply before voicing your ideas will contribute to better team communication.

- Leverage one-on-one conversations: Introverted leaders shine in one-on-one settings. Use this ability to build personal rapport with your team, understand their unique strengths, and create tailored work strategies.

- Prioritize solitude for strategic planning: As an introvert, solitude is a powerful tool for reflection and strategic planning. Use this time to think deeply about your leadership strategy and its implementation.

8.4. Navigating Challenges of Introverted Leadership

Despite the unique strengths that introverted leaders possess, there are also challenges that you may face. It is essential to acknowledge these potential obstacles and develop strategies to overcome them.

For instance, as an introverted leader, communication, especially in large group settings, can be challenging. However, this can be counteracted by understanding your communication style, embracing it, and honing it to create an impactful presence. Additionally, with the help of technology, one can effectively communicate with teams or large audiences via emails, messaging platforms, and collaborative digital boards.

Another challenge can be networking and forming professional relationships especially in new settings—an aspect that may not come naturally to introspective individuals. Rather than viewing networking as a demanding social obligation, approach it as a series of meaningful one-on-one conversations, which is a get-to-know-you session rather than a spotlight moment.

Remember, every leadership style comes with its strengths and hardships. What sets successful leaders apart is their ability to recognize these challenges and transform them into opportunities for growth.

8.5. Conclusion: Carving Your Unique Leadership Path

In the end, the most important takeaway is this: embrace your unique leadership style without seeking to fit into the extroverted leadership mold. Your reflective nature, combined with a natural propensity to listen and empathize, positions you perfectly to inspire those around you, drive change, and lead with conviction and authenticity.

Remember, the world needs more leaders like you who value deep connection over surface-level small talk, thoughtful answers over impulsive reaction, and empathetic understanding over dismissive commands. As an introverted leader, you carry within you the power to redefine leadership, and this chapter serves as a guiding light as you carve your own unique path.

Chapter 9. Communicating Effectively as an Introvert

Every ounce of this chapter is committed to carving out an understanding of communicating effectively as an introvert. Replete with profound strategies, intuitive methods, and empowering tips, this exhaustive exploration will arm you with a formidable linguistic toolkit.

9.1. The Intrinsic Value of Communication

Communication plays a crucial role in our personal, social and professional lives. It may involve an exchange of ideas, sharing thoughts or emotions, voicing concerns or simply making oneself known to the world. For introverts, this can be an arduous journey as mainstream communication styles often favor extroversion. However, being an introvert doesn't mean that effective communication is beyond your reach. It's paramount to grasp that your introverted nature can actually equip you with unique communication skills capable of culminating into meaningful connections.

9.2. Tapping into Introspection

Introspection, the cornerstone of introversion, serves as an indispensable tool for cultivating effective communication skills. As introverts, you are endowed with a capacity for deep thought, subtlety of understanding, and delicate handling of interpersonal relationships. This inherent trait allows an introvert to ruminate on their thoughts, refine their ideas, and deliver succinct and targeted messages. Inner reflection and contemplation pave the way for clarity of communication, a feature admired and respected in any conversation.

9.3. Listening: Your Strong Suit

Active listening is an aspect of communication where introverts naturally excel. It involves not only hearing the words spoken by others but also tuning into nonverbal cues, mood, and emotions. By doing so, introverts can marinate in the thoughts of others, develop an in-depth understanding, and respond more thoughtfully. This quality of active listening fosters trust, indicates respect, and engenders empathy, all of which position you as a captivating conversationalist despite your quiet demeanor.

9.4. Modulating Your Voice

Voice modulation goes beyond mere volume control; it involves varying your pitch, controlling your pace, and placing emphasis where needed to articulate your message compellingly. As an introvert, you can harness the power of voice modulation to assert your presence in group discussions, meetings, or casual chats. Given practice, this can help you achieve a rhythm that doesn't strain your natural inclinations or burn you out. It provides you the flexibility to command attention while preserving your energy.

9.5. Your Words, Your Power

Introverts often have a rich inner world filled with thoughts and ideas ready to be shared. Harnessing these thoughts carefully and delivering them with tactful eloquence can result in powerful communication. Craft your words diligently, use thoughtful pauses to build anticipation, and leverage your comfort with silence to bear your thoughts with grace. Armed with these skills, you can turn precision of language into your power.

9.6. Non-Verbal Communication: The Silent Dialogue

While verbal communication often attracts considerable attention, non-verbal communication serves as a quiet yet potent dialogue conducted in silence. Considering introverts' natural discretion and their ability to pick up subtleties, understanding and utilizing non-verbal cues such as facial expressions, eye contact, and body posture can enrich the communication process.

9.7. Introverts in Digital Communication

The digital world gives introverts an expanded playground to practice and perfect their communication skills. Email, messaging platforms, and social media channels allow you to gather your thoughts, refine your message, and respond with less immediacy but increased thoughtfulness. This shift from in-person to virtual communication offers you a platform to shine by playing to your strengths.

9.8. Communication Challenges: Struggles and Strategies

Every individual, introvert or not, encounters challenges in the spectrum of communication. However, introverts may face distinctive struggles such as speaking up in groups, asserting themselves, or dealing with interruptions. To tackle these roadblocks, strategies such as pre-planning your points, practicing assertiveness, and managing your energy can prove quite beneficial.

9.9. Find Your Unique Voice

Ultimately, effective communication for introverts is about finding and refining your unique voice. Embrace the elements that make your way of communication unique and valuable, harness them, and present them to the world. This is not about imitation or a cookie-cutter approach but about showcasing your authentic self. Because just as this world needs extroverted communicators, it just as much needs the thoughtful, introspective voices of introverts like you.

To sum up, effective communication is not limited to those who talk more or louder. As an introvert, you can use your inherent strengths like deep introspection, quality listening, and precise articulation to your advantage. By recognizing the potent power within you and embracing yourself as you are, you can not only thrive but lead in the realm of communication.

Chapter 10. Building Relationships: Networking for Introverts

An integral part of thriving in an extroverted world is building relationships, an arena often deemed as challenging by introverts. Nonetheless, forming robust, meaningful relationships and networking doesn't need to be an uphill battle for those of us with more introverted personalities. We must understand that networking, for introverts, is not about amassing countless contacts; instead, it's about deep, more meaningful connections.

10.1. The Power of One-on-One Connections

Introverts are masters of one-on-one connections; they thrive in environments that facilitate in-depth dialogues instead of boisterous group discussions. Multiple studies have confirmed the power of individual conversation, noting that they can lead to more significant outcomes, such as the formation of deep emotional connections or even partnerships. When you're networking as an introvert, aim for these smaller interactions. Invite someone you're interested in learning from out for coffee, or propose a one-on-one lunch to foster alignment with a colleague.

10.2. The Importance of Active Listening and Observation

One strategy introverts excel at that gives them a unique edge in networking is their propensity for listening and observation. Introverts are often more comfortable taking in their surroundings and paying close attention to verbal and non-verbal cues from conversation partners. This ability is invaluable in relationship-building. By practicing active listening, we demonstrate respect and interest, which in turn fuels deeper conversations and stronger connections.

10.3. Authenticity in Building Relationships

Another strong suit of introverted individuals is their authenticity. It's no secret that people are drawn to those who are real and honest, and this authenticity adds to the appeal of introverts in networking scenarios. Rather than putting on a show or emulating a persona, remaining true to your nature and upholding your values can be the most effective networking tool. People appreciate and trust authenticity; it fosters a sense of reliability and, subsequently, more meaningful relationships.

10.4. Leveraging Digital Platforms

In the digital era, there's a myth that introverts are anti-technology. Nothing could be further from the truth. The online world provides ample opportunities to build relationships without the pressure of face-to-face interaction. Whether it be through LinkedIn, virtual conferences, online forums, or mentorship platforms, the digital space allows for a more controlled and thoughtful networking approach that suits introverts very well. However, keep in mind the importance of maintaining a balance between online and offline networking to ensure a wider and more dynamic network.

10.5. Strategizing and Preparing for Networking Events

Lastly, the idea of attending networking events can be daunting for introverts. However, with careful planning and strategy, these occasions can be navigated smoothly. For instance, setting a goal for the number of people you want to meet or the kinds of discussions you want to have can lend purpose to your networking efforts. Additionally, researching attendees and preparing questions or topics of discussion beforehand can boost your confidence and help in generating productive conversations.

Each of these strategies forms a cornerstone of the introvert's networking guide. Armed with these, introverts can defy stereotypes and leverage their unique strengths to build lifelong connections. So, whenever you find yourself questioning your ability to connect with others, remember that your introverted personality is not a hindrance but a strength. It provides you with a unique, thoughtful, and authentic approach to connecting with others that is rare and deeply valued. To reiterate, always keep in mind that being an introvert is not about having fewer connections, but rather about having more profound ones.

Chapter 11. Embracing Extraversion: Striking the Balance

In the world of personality types, it may initially seem as though introverts and extroverts exist on two opposite ends of a spectrum. From the way we recharge our psychological energy to the nature of our interactions with others, introverts and extroverts may display stark differences. However, as insightful as the binary concept of introversion and extroversion can be, it does not provide a comprehensive understanding of the complexities and nuances of human behavior. Factually, we are all ambiverts to some extent, embodying characteristics from both ends of the continuum.

11.1. Embracing Ambiversion: Blurring the Lines

Let's begin by shattering the myth that introversion and extraversion are mutually exclusive traits. The majority of us fall somewhere in between introversion and extroversion, in a state often referred to as 'ambiversion.' Ambiversion implies a blend of the characteristics of both types, maintaining a healthy balance between inward-focused and outward-focused energies.

This equilibrium enables us to adapt to a multitude of social contexts and to develop multifaceted personas. The key lies in understanding that we are not constrained by a label, but have the ability to exhibit an array of behaviors based on the situation. Embracing ambiversion signifies legitimizing the introverted aspects of oneself and acknowledging the need for intermittent engagement with extroverted activities, tailored to our own unique configurations of comfort and challenge.

11.2. Understanding Extraversion: Catering to Your Needs

To balance the introverted aspects of your personality, it's essential to build an understanding of what extraversion is, and in particular, the aspects that can be comfortably adopted into your lifestyle. Extraversion, in its essence, is often characterized by a preference for social interaction, action orientation, and assertiveness.

However, adopting aspects of extraversion does not imply radically changing who you are or defying your inner nature. It's about developing a finer tune to interact with a largely extroverted world. You may adopt extroverted strategies for presenting yourself or honing your communication without suppressing your profound introspective qualities.

11.3. Approachable Extraverted Activities: Entrance of the Comfort Zone

There are several ways in which introverts can begin to integrate extroverted elements into their lifestyle, knowingly expanding their comfort zone. Establish a habit of occasionally stepping into social events. This does not necessarily mean you start frequenting boisterous parties. Rather, it could be something as unassuming as joining a book club, attending an artistic workshop, or registering for a community event related to an area of interest.

Another method might be to gradually increase your interactions with colleagues or friends. Again, this is not a call to engage in incessant chitchat, but an encouragement to express your thoughts or ideas during shared moments. Remember, these activities should not drain your energy but should challenge you in a balanced manner.

11.4. Creating a Healthy Social Balance: Truly Recharging

Recognizing and protecting your introvert energy is crucial for successfully integrating extroverted elements into your life, creating a healthy balance. Practice tuning into your own needs and reactions, taking time for yourself when you need it, and embracing solitude to recharge after periods of social interaction. This reinforcing cycle ensures your energy resources are maintained, keeping you resilient and capable of showing up in the world as your best self.

11.5. Leveraging These Elements: Achieving the Optimal Balance

Finally, the art of embracing extraversion as an introvert lies in leveraging these elements in a way that complements your intrinsic qualities. Maintain an active dialogue with yourself to identify what actions and environments feel most comfortable and productive. Gradually leaning into extroverted practices ensures the creation of a lifestyle that balances the needs and strengths of both introverted and extroverted aspects of your personality.

The chapter does not end here, but is more of a starting point on your journey to find and strike an optimal balance. The objective is not to completely transform yourself into an extrovert, but rather to become a versatile ambivert. So, experiment, reflect and adapt, as you develop a balanced lifestyle that cherishes the introverted core of your being, while also harnessing the dynamic energy of extraversion.